Mastering the Practice of ZEN

The Key to Living a More Peaceful Life

RON KNESS

By reading this document, the reader agrees that under no circumstances are we responsible for any losses, direct or indirect, which are incurred as a result of the use of information contained within this document, including, but not limited to, —errors, omissions, or inaccuracies.

This book is for **personal use only**.

ISBN: 9781795704953

Contents

Introduction

A Zen lifestyle is an attempt to lead a simpler life. To do so effectively, you will need to take on a set of habits that minimize, simplify and sort out the chaos of your everyday life.

By incorporating Zen habits into your everyday routine, you can learn to focus on what's meaningful in life and give all your attention to that focus. At the same time, you will also hone your skills to a razor-sharp edge remove the unwanted and unimportant stuff from life. The goal is to lead a simpler yet more purposeful and productive life.

This book will help you get started with Zen fundamentals and how to implement these habits into your life.

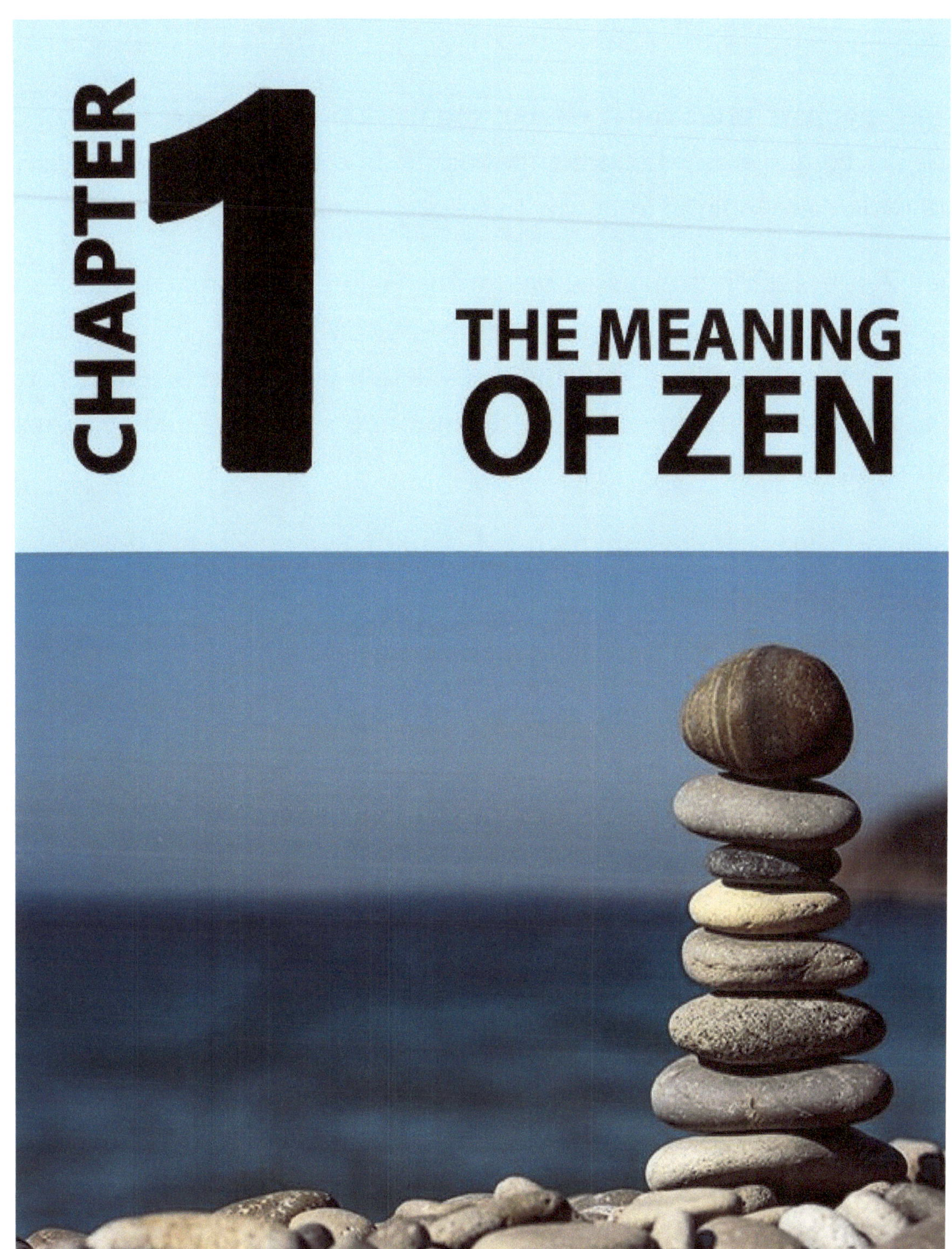

CHAPTER
1
THE MEANING
OF ZEN

Chapter 1 - The Meaning of ZEN

You may not have practiced it yet, but you most probably have heard of Zen. It is a common word making the rounds in different circles, primarily where people are looking for a way to simplify their lives.

In fact, Zen has often been associated with certain aspects like tranquility, mindfulness, concentration and anything else that can help restore some order in today's fast-paced and chaotic lives that we live. In essence, Zen tries to understand the meaning of life without being distracted by logical or rational thought.

The practice does demand an intense discipline which, when followed properly, will let you get better at dodging distractions. But this is easier said than done. If you come from the western part of the hemisphere where intellectual thinking and multitasking dominate, it can be challenging to adapt to Zen.

The Origins of Zen

Historically, Zen has been practiced for centuries in Oriental monasteries by monks and goes by various names. For instance, the Chinese refer to it as *Ch'an*, the Vietnamese as *Thien* and the Koreans as *Seon*. But it is the Japanese rendering of this aspect of Buddhism that is known as Zen.

Zen Buddhism was brought to China by the Indian monk, Bodhidharma sometime in the 6th century. Then, it became known as Ch'an and then spread to Korea and Japan. Under the sixth Chinese patriarch, Huineng, Zen shed many of its inherent Indian trappings becoming more Chinese. It also became more of the Zen that we now think of.

But it was not until the middle of the 20th century that Zen Buddhism became popular in the West.

Zen, as we know it today is a way of living where people find happiness and peace within themselves. They learn to be more aware of their surroundings and the present rather than be distracted by an influx of information overkill. Zen teaches individuals how to lead a more disciplined and simple life instead of a contrived and artificial one.

So if you are looking for a way to incorporate more Zen into your life then read on. Here is a quick rundown of what to do and not do in your life as you start your Zen journey.

What to Do?

At its very basic, Zen teaches you to be fully aware and live in each moment. This means you should work with a single-pointed awareness.

For instance, if you're cleaning, then you're fully present for the act of cleaning alone. If you're spending time with family, they are your only focus and nothing else. Or if you're relaxing at home, then you're not thinking about the day's events or worrying about tomorrow.

Keeping things simple and focused also lets you understand that less is more. So while you may be doing less, you're actually giving it your everything, and coming out with a more gratified experience.

Keeping things minimal will also help you figure out what's important and unimportant in life. In a way, it's decluttering your everyday affairs. But decluttering here doesn't only refer to your physical life as in dealing with everyday activities and chores, but also decluttering your thoughts.

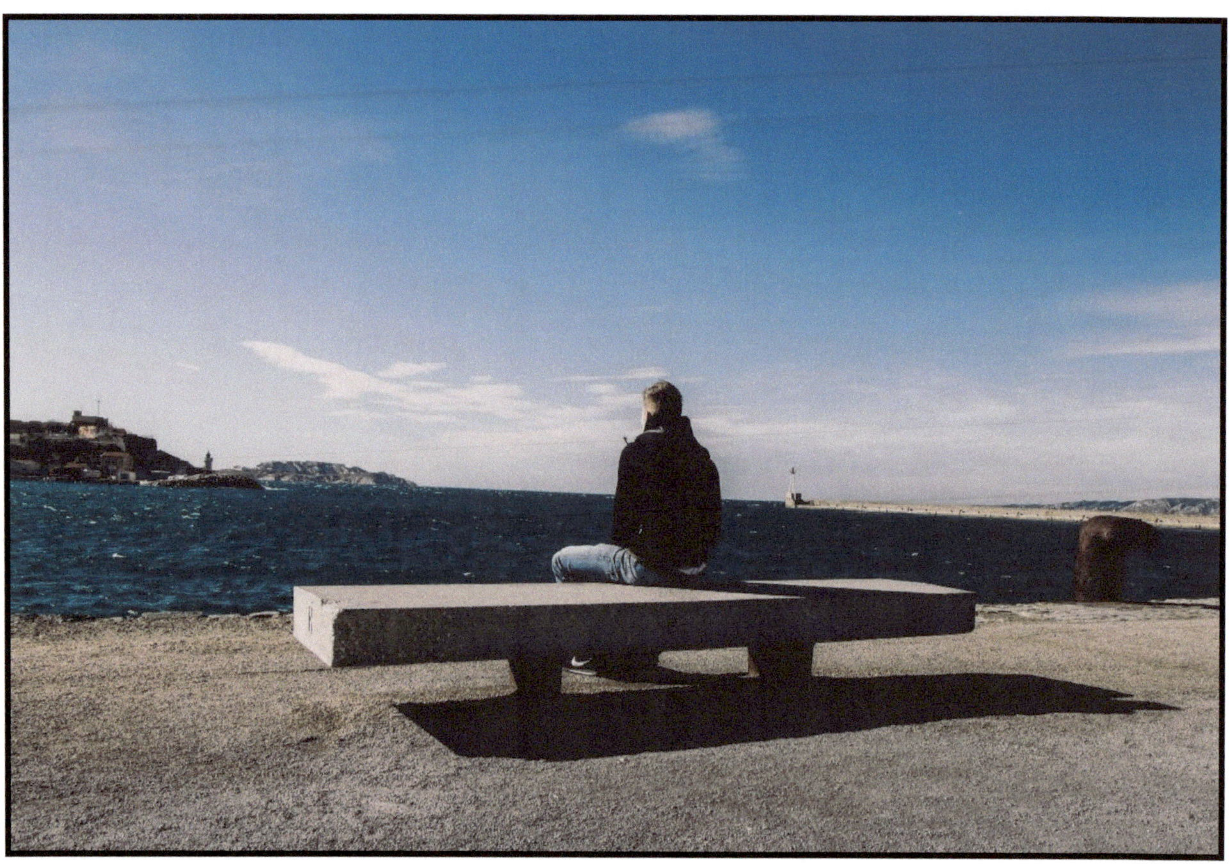

Often times, you get caught up in conflicting or confusing thoughts which can really affect your state of mind. As such, you become distracted, absent-minded, and even distraught. This, in turn, shows up in your behavior possibly making you fearful, troubled and preoccupied. You need to rid yourself of all this to lead a Zen life.

Then there is your attachment to your goals and dreams. Now, this is not a bad thing as long as you work towards it positively. But if you reach a point where you convince yourself that you can't be happy without it, then you're in trouble.

This kind of attachment is not healthy at all. Unfortunately, many people fall victim to this mentality. To enter the Zen zone in your life, you need to answer a few questions first.

Ask yourself why you're pursuing your goal. Is it because you believe you'll find happiness? Or is it something that will let you help others? Perhaps, you consider it worth spending your time on?

Now look on the flip side and see what this pursuit is costing you in terms of your own wellbeing or the wellbeing of others. If you find telling yourself that you'll be happy when... (you achieve your goal), that itself is stopping you from enjoying the moment.

Anything that stops you from living in the moment also holds you back from realizing happiness and peace in that very same moment.

So to truly experience a Zen life, you need to work both on your body and your mind. On a physical level, practices like breathing, smiling more, and meditation can all help calm down the chaos in life. But the same can also have a surprisingly calming effect on your mind.

If the chaos in your physical life is levelled, then your state of mind will also relax.

What Not to Do?

Just as it's important to know what steps to follow when adopting a Zen lifestyle, it's equally important to know what not to do as well.

You need to find peace with yourself first before you can proceed onto anything else. And to do that you need to be happy with who you are. In other words, you can say that you need to get to like yourself better first.

How do you do that? Here's how.

For starters, you need to stop comparing yourself or your situation to others. When you compare, you sabotage your happiness and start to feel lacking.

Negative thoughts like what you have (or don't have) start to creep up and you make yourself suffer for no reason. You need to stop that right away.

That said, you also need to stop judging. Judging never feels good because judgement is a heavy burden.

Another thing you may want to work on is worry. If you want to adopt Zen habits for a healthier, more peaceful lifestyle, you should cut down on worrying about everything. Oftentimes, worry stems from fear or an urge to feel in control. If you sense that you're starting to lose control, you begin to worry.

This is exactly what doesn't work in a Zen lifestyle. Worrying only creates a negative energy within yourself and around you. And with a troubled head on your shoulders, you won't be able to focus on the moment.

The do's and don'ts of Zen are a mixed bag. Some are straightforward and quick while others are more of a work-in-progress. But in the long run, if you follow these steps consistently, they will come together and change your life in a big way.

CHAPTER 2

DON'T FORGET TO BREATHE

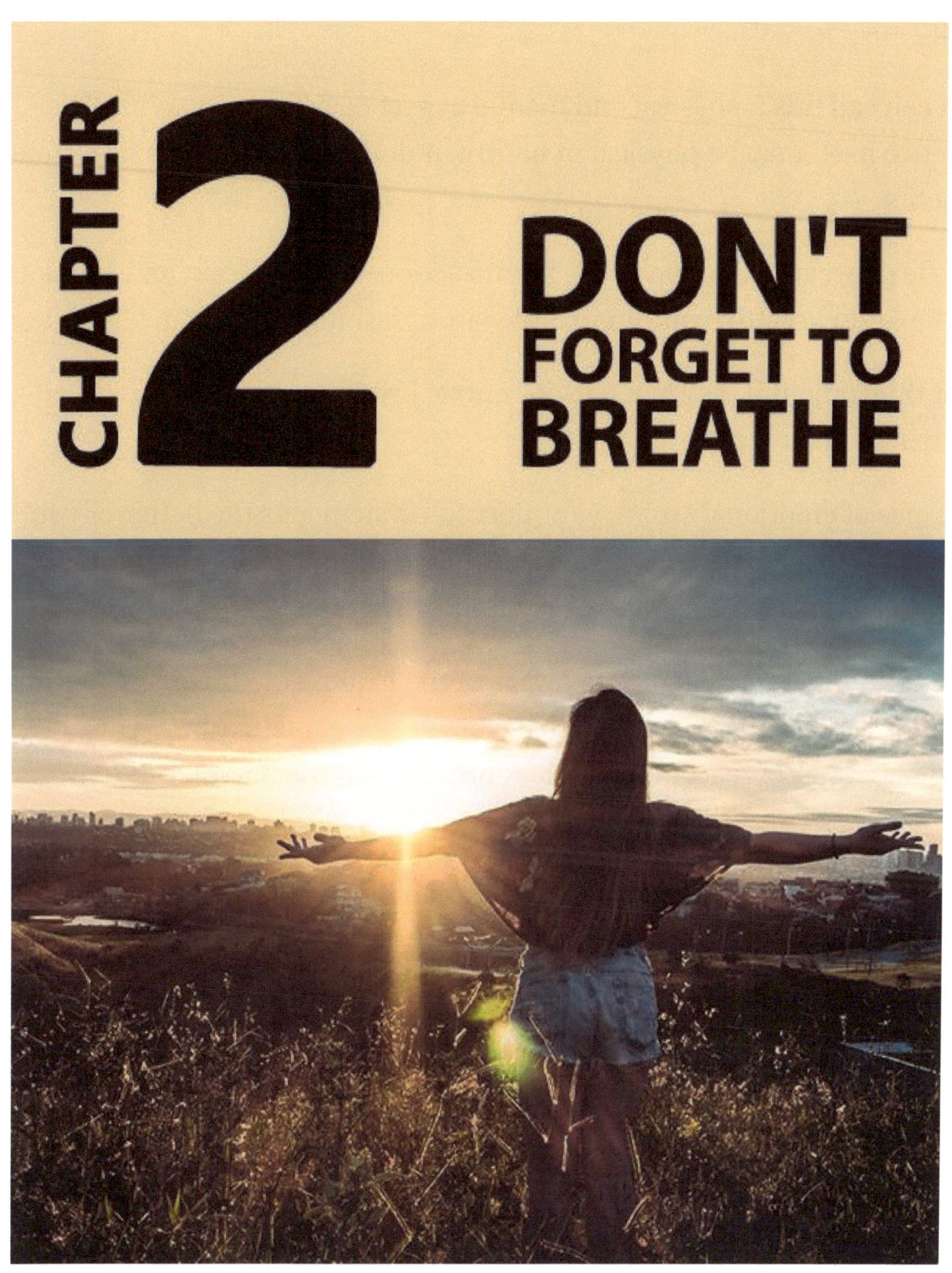

Chapter 2 - Don't Forget to Breathe

You can call this a physical and mental aspect of Zen habits. While the practice itself may be physical in nature, it does have truly amazing mental benefits.

Physical, because it involves the innate actions of inhalation and exhalation. And mental because your mind and your breathing rate are always linked.

Just think about it, a rapid, out-of-control breath results in a rapid, out-of-control mind or vice versa.

In times of emotional stress, your nervous system gets the better of you. This leads to an increase in heart rate and tense muscles. Your breathing becomes rapid and this impacts your body overall.

However, not many people are aware of the healing qualities that breathing holds. Your breath can be used to deal with these fluctuations. This, in turn, results in muscle relaxation and less pressure on the nervous system.

On the other hand, when your breathing is calm and controlled, so is your mind. Here is how controlled breathing can help you achieve a Zen life.

Breathing for Relaxation

Have you ever tried taking a really deep breath? Try it and you will feel more relaxed and less anxious right away. I have found that by breathing in deeply through my nose for four seconds, holding it for four and exhaling through my mouth for eight seconds, I can drop my heartrate by at least four to six beats per minute.

You have no idea how powerful your breath is. Making breathing exercises part of your life can bring about significant improvement not only in your quality of breath, but also the quality of life. You will feel increased vibrancy and clarity that you may have been missing out on for years.

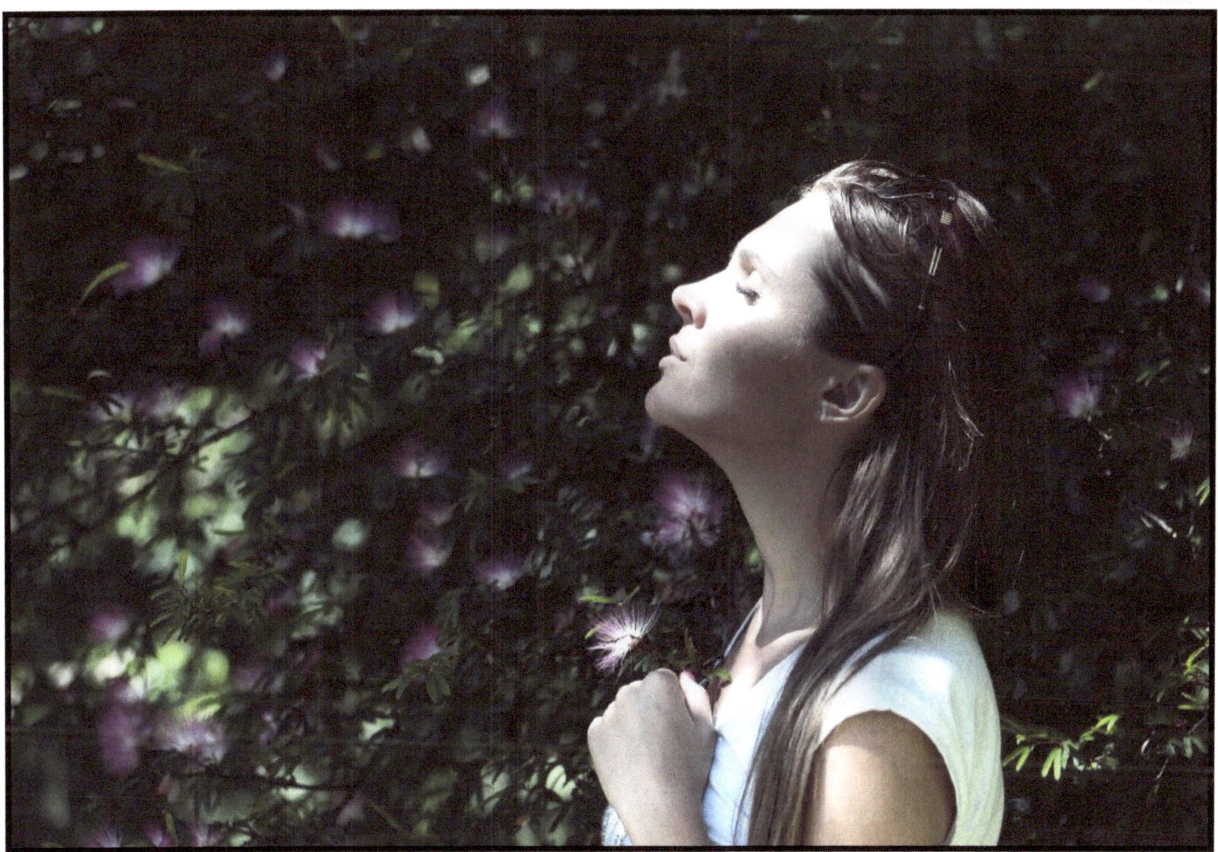

When practicing breathing, opt for calm breathing. Calm breathing basically involves breathing slowly and is very effective. It reduces physical symptoms such as panic attacks and anxiety. This is a therapy that can be practiced anywhere, anytime. With this technique, when you breathe to relax you actually teach yourself stress management.

And the importance of a calm and controlled mind in Zen habits cannot be undermined. Even people who don't have a Zen lifestyle have been learning to control their breath for a long time.

That's because it has long been a method of calming the mind in yoga and meditation. And now it's even being used to quell anxiety and curb panic attacks in medical and psychiatric practices.

In essence, controlled breathing helps clear the mind and body of negativity. The same also activates the mind and soul. Ancient yogis have spent ages practicing and refining optimal breathing techniques. To them, breathing is the easiest and most natural way to release stress. And it can be your best way too!

The Benefits

Breathing for relaxation holds massive benefits. There are many on a physical level such as detoxification. In fact, when you breathe, your body potentially releases about 70% of toxins it holds inside.

Correct exhalation releases optimal carbon dioxide which also rids the body of toxins. As this constant state of detox takes place, your mind also clears out and you feel better.

In another area, breathing acts as a masseuse for your organs. The stomach, liver, pancreas all receives massage therapy when you breathe. The continuous movements of the diaphragm and abdomen during breathing allows circulation to improve and studies state that breathing helps strengthen muscles.

Proper oxygen supply also helps reduce the burden on the heart. When you breathe properly you make your lungs more efficient. The lungs start receiving more oxygen which benefits the heart. This reduces pressure on the heart to deliver oxygen to the tissues.

On its benefits for the mind, proper breathing helps reduce tension, relaxes the mind and can even elevate your mood.

You know that when you're in a state of anger, your body tightens and tenses and your breathing becomes shallow. As this happens, the supply of oxygen to the body diminishes. But learning to breathe correctly allows the oxygen to properly reach all parts of the body.

Likewise, breathing properly has even been connected to reducing the formation of clots. When you breathe purposefully, you allow tightened spots to soften. When this happens, you are able to bring clarity as the body is relaxed.

You are also aware that when the mind is at ease you feel less emotional. With a content state of mind, there is a sense of strength that the body surpasses. In this way, breathing helps reduce emotional stress and the uneasy feelings that come with it.

So many of these effects of mindful breathing will make your Zen lifestyle even more effective. You know by now that when your mind is in tranquil state, your body will respond likewise. So here are a few techniques to relax you mind and body.

Zen Breathing Techniques

The Complete Yogi Breath

The principle behind this technique is to fill up your entire abdomen and chest with air. Fresh air should enter your body like a new life force and renew it. This internal process also stretches your spine, tones internal organs, and improves circulation throughout the body.

To do this, exhale completely so that everything hollows out. Following a short pause, inhale deeply. As you inhale feel your belly expand outward. Next, move your focus to your lower back and sides, filling them with air.

Once you've filled these with air, shift your focus to your ribcage filling the midsection of your abdomen. Allow your ribs to puff out.

Finally, fill your upper chest area all the way to your collarbones. This should also lift your heart as you come into a tall posture. This entire inhale may be done in a few quick seconds or stretched to an extended period of 15 or so seconds.

For the exhale, keep your chest lifted and your posture tall. Starting with the belly first, exhale and empty the belly. Then move toward your spine and empty the midsection. Round off the exhale with emptying the chest. Ideally, your exhale should be longer than your inhale or at least of equal length.

Bellows Breath

Inspired by yoga and other meditation techniques, this method can help improve alertness, clarify your mind and make you energetic.

If you feel lazy, hazy, or as if you're moving in slow motion, try this breathing technique.

Sitting up tall, relax your shoulders and take a few deep breaths in and out from your nose. Begin the bellows breath by exhaling through your nose. Follow by inhaling through the nose once again.

This practice should ensure that your breath comes from your diaphragm. As you breathe in and out, make sure to keep your head, neck, shoulders and chest absolutely still.

Complete one cycle of 10 breaths followed by a 15-30 second break. Start the next round with 20 breaths. Break and then do a final round of 30 bellows breaths.

This practice is best done first thing in the morning when you need to start your day off right. You can also do this during your mid-day slump or right before a workout session.

Breath Counting

This is a simple technique used in Zen practices to calm an active mind.

Start with abdominal inhales and exhales. At the end of the first exhale, make a mental note saying "one". Inhale, exhale and mentally count "two". Continue breathing until you reach "ten".

Next start counting backwards until you reach "one". The point here is to keep track of the numbers so that your attention stays put and doesn't detract.

This exercise is a strength building one for the mind. It removes distracting thoughts and builds concentration power. So if you've never given much thought to your breathing, now's the time to get started.

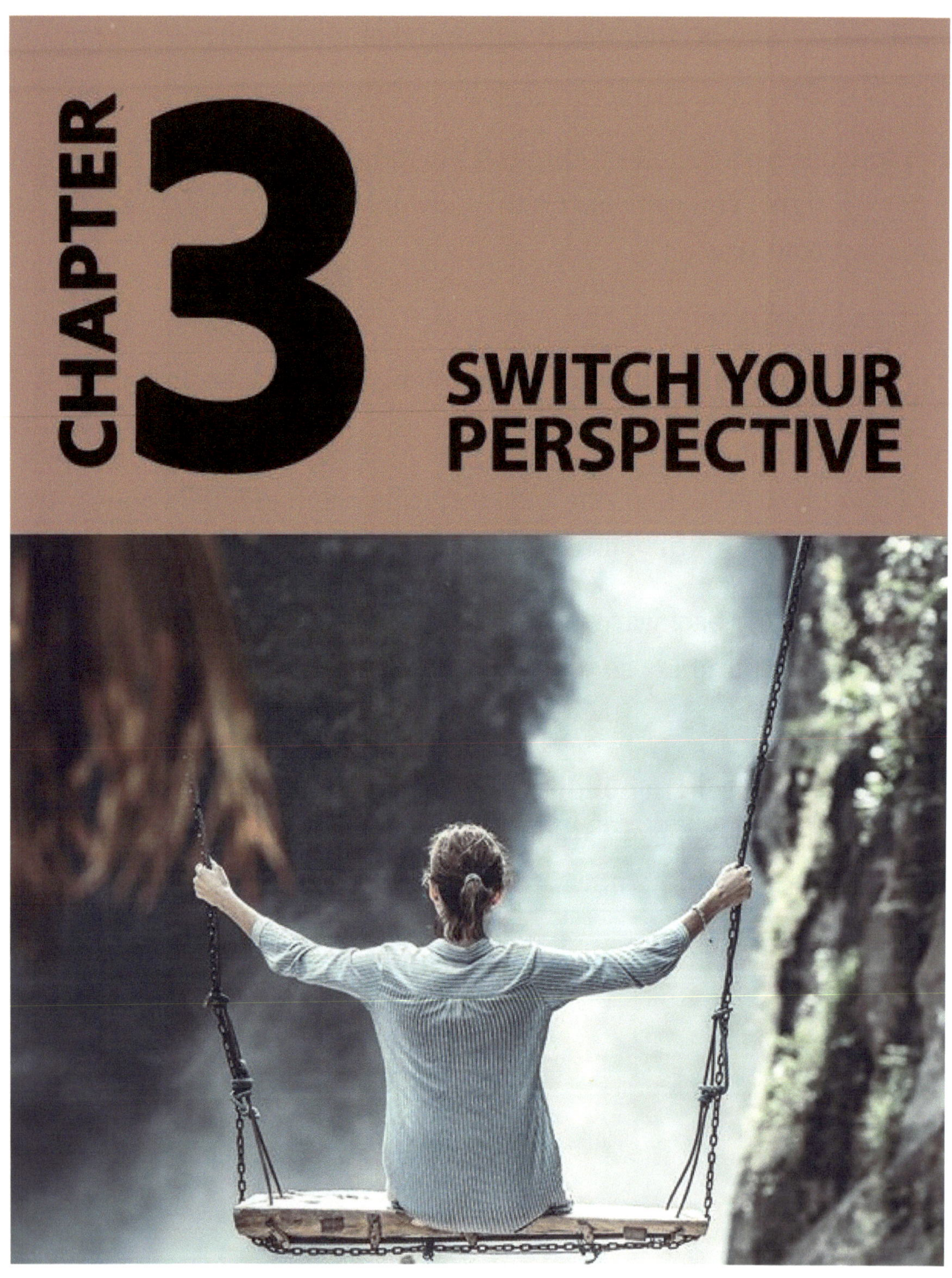
CHAPTER
3
SWITCH YOUR PERSPECTIVE

Chapter 3 - Switch Your Perspective

Oftentimes, people feel that their focus is not under their control. You may have had the same suspicions about yourself.

But the truth is that what you focus on is what you experience. If you spend too much time focusing on things you don't need, your mind gets caught in a web. You try to multitask, switch from one thing to the next, or simply end up putting things off. Actually, we can't multitask. In reality our mind switches quickly from one thing to another making it appear you are doing more than one thing at a time, but you are not.

And with time, it becomes hard to break out of the habit of switching and being distracted all the time.

However, the simple truth is that your happiness depends on the way you think and how you respond to the environment you live in. Perspective has a huge role to play when it comes to your happiness.

So how do you train your mind to stay more focused and how can you switch your perspective?

Here are some steps you can take to do so.

Stay with One Thing at a Time

Too many people are guilty of doing too many things at the same time. When you demand your attention to jump from one thing to another, you will have a busy, fractured, and most likely unproductive day.

Switching tasks frequently requires a supreme level of functioning, meaning that you must use a lot of brain power and energy even before you start a task. No wonder it ends up draining your effectiveness.

Zen teaches you to do the exact opposite. With Zen habits in your life, you will choose a task that needs doing and then stick with it. A good starting point may be to ask why this particular task is important for you. If you can give yourself a good enough reason why this task means more than others, then that's where you need to start.

As you start your task, shift all your attention to it. Shut out any distractions and clear your mind. Don't think about or start doing something else until you have finished what you started. Train yourself to focus on the task at hand and resist the urge to look elsewhere.

This practice will keep you steadily grounded in the present and let you give your best to whatever task you choose to do.

This rule is applicable to even the simplest of things. For instance, when you eat, just eat. When you pour water, just do that. When you go walking, just walk.

In instances where you may have to move onto something else, at least put away the unfinished task to return to later.

Taking it slow in this way doesn't mean you're being lazy. What it does mean is that you're doing it right. You may be doing less, but you're doing it well.

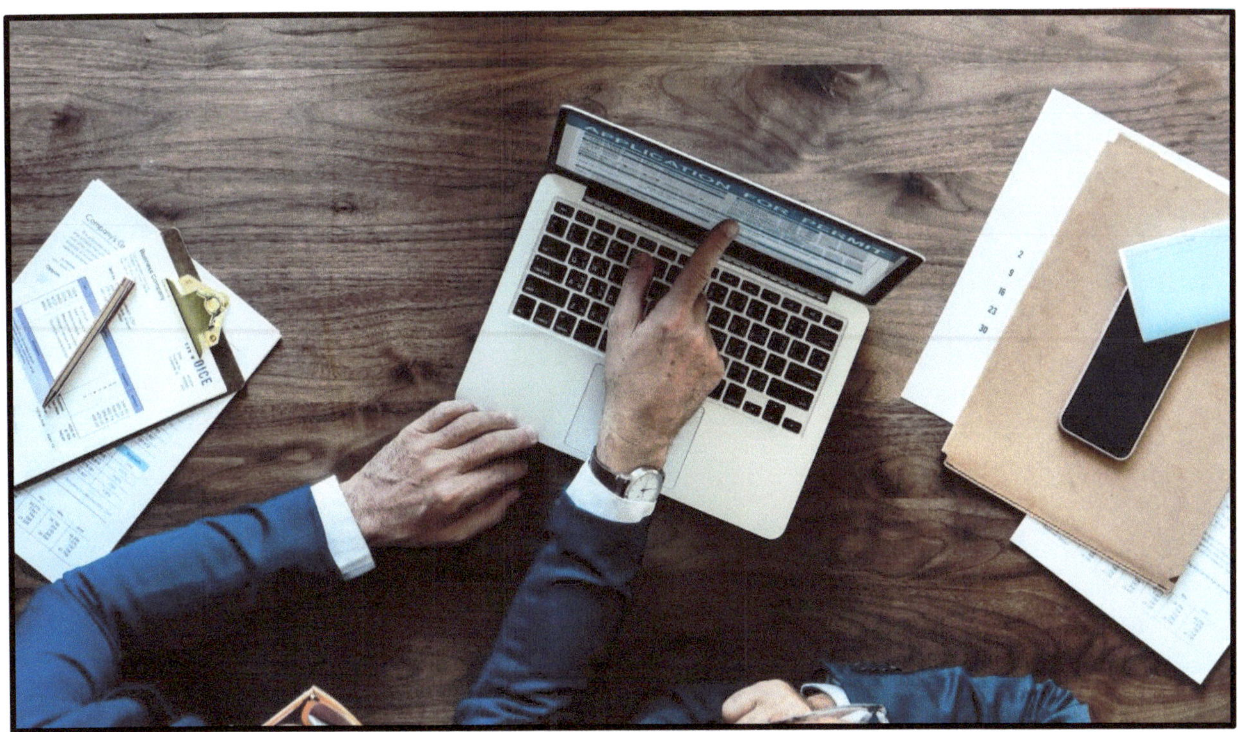

Sometimes, you'll have to deal with everyday distractions, like the digital world for instance. In fact, there is now a lot of research pointing to the fact that digital distractions are making people not only dumb but also twitchy.

Not only does this concern stop you from concentrating, it also stops you from resting, both of which are equally damaging.

Focus on the Process

Changing perspective requires your focus. You can't adopt a positive life if you are constantly distracted and losing focus on important matters.

 Focusing on the process and how things should be dealt with will make you wiser. It's worth to mention that it's incredibly important that instead of focusing on the outcome, learn to focus on the process. This will help you in quite a few different ways.

For instance, focusing on the process will eliminate external factors. What this means is that decisions based on outcomes often end up using wrong techniques.

But when you focus on how to get things done, you are better able to polish your skills. As you work your way through something, you realize the pitfalls and also discover ways to remediate the problems.

Plus, focusing on the process also lets you enjoy the moment. You become more engaged in the present and at what you're doing. And you will do it better too.

Another perk of focusing on the process rather than the outcome is that you get more control over what you're doing.

In other words, you don't have control over the outcome, but you do have control over the process. When you give something your best, the outcome is likely to be good as well.

If anything, focusing on the process will make you more confident in learning new skills. These skills will make you better at decision making. You will have fewer worries about the future, and your focus will be on the present.

To better focus on the process, engage in only one thing at a time. Do the work slowly and deliberately. (This doesn't mean lazily, only that you need to take your time and move purposefully).

When doing so, make your actions deliberate instead of random. There is also a need to put space between things.

What this means is that try not to schedule things too close together but leave some gaps in between. This will give you a more relaxed structure to work with. It will also provide some wiggle room if one task takes longer than expected.

The whole point of Zen is to enjoy what you're doing, so try not to rush through your life.

Don't Rationalize

Rationalization is defined as something where you apparently come up with rational explanations for certain behaviors. The point is to make that behavior seem optimal even when it's not.

However, the same definition could also lead you to conclude that rationalization, essentially, is the act of making excuses. Either way, rationalizing doesn't always help which is why you need to avoid it.

When you want to incorporate Zen habits into your life, you need to stop making excuses.

As you've seen earlier, Zen does require a certain degree of discipline. So while missing one day of meditation won't derail your progress much, making it a habit certainly can.

The biggest problem with skip-days like these is that they eventually lead to quitting or giving up. The one-time exception then becomes the rule.

Getting off track can make it very difficult to get back on track. That's why Zen encourages establishing a daily routine as we will see in an upcoming chapter.

For now, let's talk a bit amore about rationalization.

You use rationalization when you try to justify less than optimal behavior or feelings. So what you're doing is finding a way to distort facts to make things appear better than they actually are.

Here's something to think about- you say you're going to follow a diet plan but that only lasts the first three days. Or you have every intention of going to the gym, since you got a membership, but only do it once.

So what happens here? A few possibilities could be that you aren't serious about it, you forget why it's important or it becomes too difficult. You may also give up in disappointment or you start to rationalize.

When something becomes difficult, your mind rationalizes telling you it's okay if you skip something once, or it's okay to have just one more (since you worked so hard for it). While this may all sound reasonable, it starts to sabotage your plans. And once you start believing these rationalizations, sticking to anything becomes next to impossible.

CHAPTER 4

SIMPLIFY YOUR LIFE

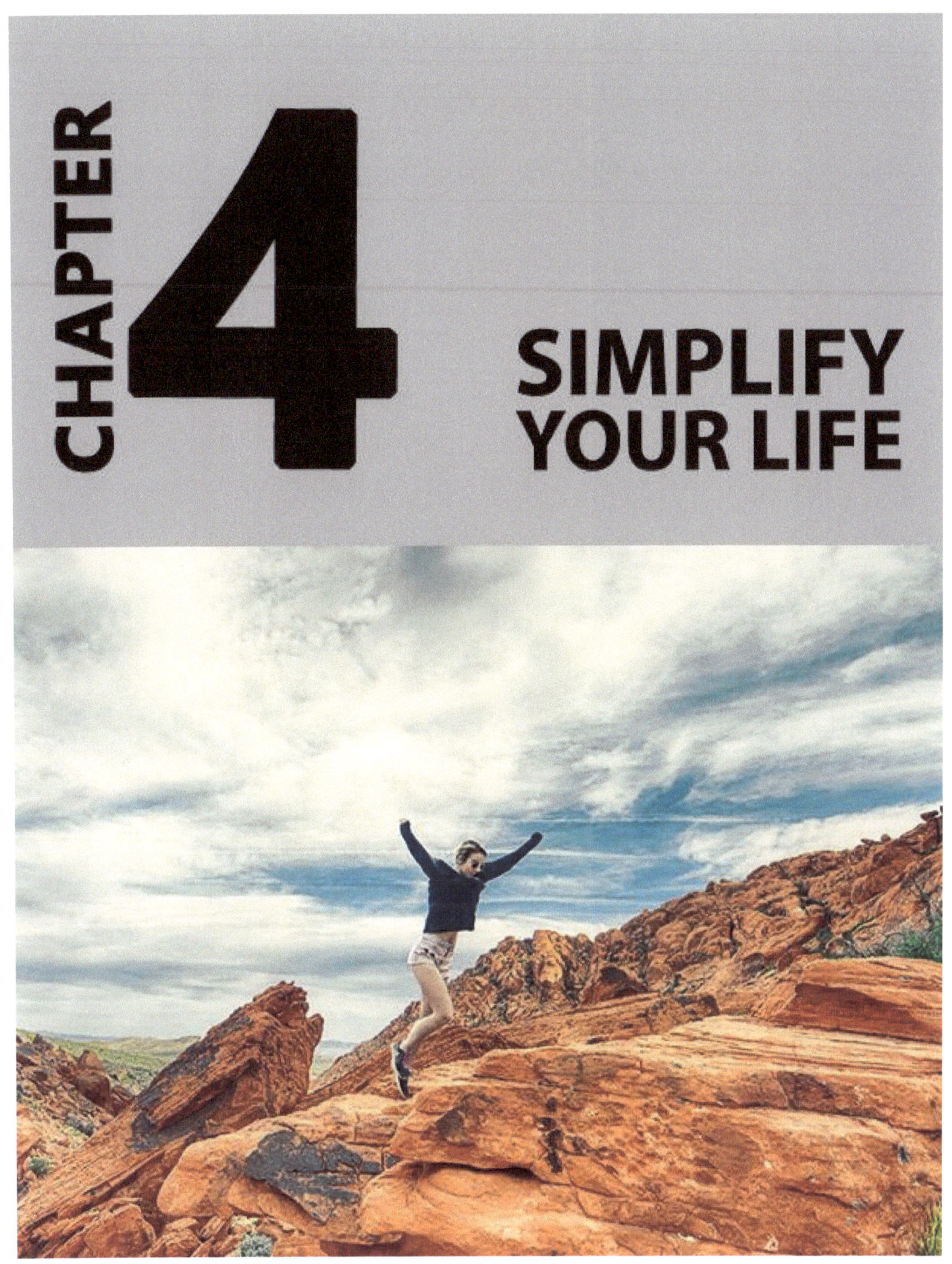

Chapter 4 - Simplify Your Life

The world you live in today exposes you to many complications. At times you end up complicating life because of overthinking. Otherwise, you end up overspending, overworking or even overcommitting.

All in all, it's an effort to get too many things done in a short amount of time. Overdoing anything also complicates things while Zen tries to teach you how to keep life simple.

If you want to have a happy life you must learn the art of simplification. Going back to its original philosophy, this simply means keeping only the important things part of your life and removing the rest.

If you think about your material possessions, getting rid of unwanted or unused stuff will certainly clear your space. This will give you peace of mind and make you happy to have a clean and open house to live in. (Try not to fill it in with more unnecessary stuff, for that just kills the idea of simplification).

But when you take the same idea to another level, simplifying life can also help you get through dark times. When you clear your mind of negativity, and unruly thoughts that don't matter, you also provide space to your mind. This space will help you absorb things that are actually important. Clear out your mind by taking in only what keeps it fresh.

Say, if you're a book collector and keep on stocking books endlessly, there will come a time when you'll run out of space. You'll either have to stop buying new books or chuck out some old ones.

Similarly, if you keep on adding unnecessary stress and things to your life there will also come a time when you'll collapse. On the other hand, if you choose to select only what is important, you'll feel weightless and happier. How you want your life to be happy depends completely on your own choices.

Here's another example to consider. Suppose you keep holding on to a grudge and dislike for someone. In the end, you'll only be wasting your time and energy dwelling over possible scenarios that might never take place. The only way you can overcome all this is to simplify your life by letting go of things that don't matter. Get rid of your emotional baggage now, your you will never actually experience Zen!

Prioritize

Once again, let's start off with a reminder of what's most important to you. Make this your unequivocal priority and stick to it.

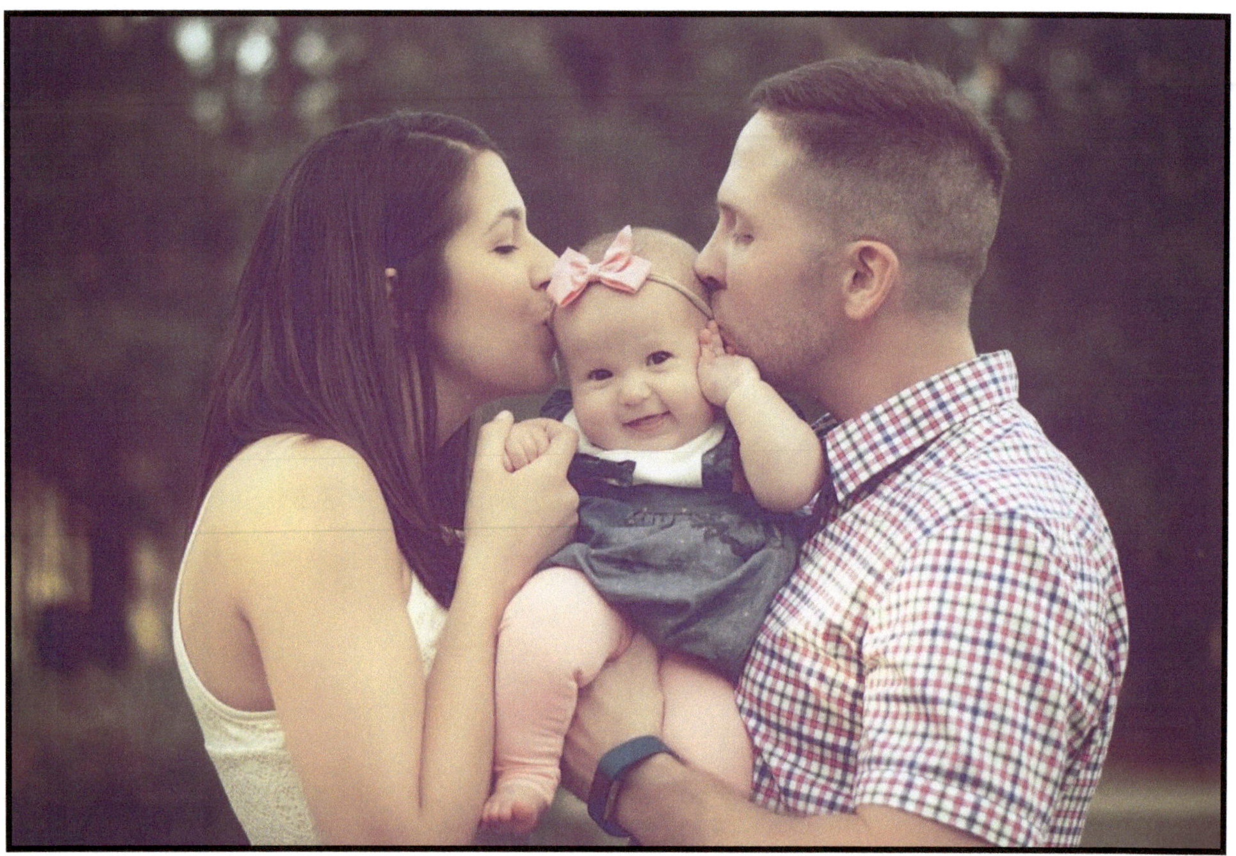

Ideally, the structure of your daily life should reflect your priorities. If you say that family is your priority, then make a commitment to spend a designated time with your spouse and kids. If you say health is a priority, then you should be doing everything you can for a healthier you. Are you truly staying away from bad/tempting foods and getting your daily dose of exercise? Or are your other commitments getting in the way?

When you prioritize, you need to be honest with yourself. What do you truly desire and what is standing your way? If you can honestly answer these two questions, you can start simplifying your life fairly easily.

As you prioritize, you'll also be filtering out a lot of excess baggage. In other words, you'll be simplifying your life.

It can become a process where you rearrange your life so that it closely reflects your priorities. If you long to spend more quality time with your kids and other significant half, then streamline your emails, put away your phone or even cut back on your work hours.

If you really want to paint, then clear out your room and make a studio space for yourself. Once you have prioritized your concerns, move on to the next step.

Declutter

When you think "declutter", you're thinking about physical as well as mental space.

This is a process of purging where you get rid of everything that is meaningless in life, or no longer offers a utility. You can start small by allotting 15-20 minutes of your day decluttering a chosen corner of your house. It could be a shelf or a cabinet. Stop after 15 minutes and come back to it the next day.

Or you could assign one entire morning to clean out your pantry or wardrobe and get it over with. You can go with whichever method works for you best.

As you purge, assign three boxes labelled "trash", "keep" and "maybe. The first two should be simple enough if you follow this advice - anything that you haven't used in the last year can go. You probably won't use it in the next year either. Keep it if you use it all the time and it still has some years left in it.

The "maybe" stash can be a bit tricky, but don't let it overwhelm you. This should be for things about which you're on the fence. Keep the box out of sight, and if you don't use it in the next six months, toss it out as well. The trick for success in decluttering is to be merciless.

The less stuff you have, the fewer distractions there will be and the simpler your life. You'll see that one of the things that give you true peace of mind is a clean, simple house.

When you talk about decluttering your mind, you'll notice that overthinking exposes your mind to blockage. Because of overload at times, you are unable to think properly. You need to deal with this quickly as it won't allow you to be happy for long.

A blocked mind becomes unaware of anything happening around it. The stream of clutter you've accumulated will turn your mental space into a chaotic mess. And soon enough, just like your closets and your cabinets, you mind needs tidying up as well.

If you're not sure about what kind of mental clutter is holding you back, just think about these things:

- Worrying about the future
- Ruminating about the past
- Thinking of everyday routines
- Complaints and grudges
- Regrets
- Commitments

If these thoughts are constantly on your mind, you need to clean out some headspace.

For starters, not everything needs attention. What's happened in the past is done, can't be undone, so why keep it around. Sure, you can and should learn from those situations, but there is not reason to hold onto them as they are just taking up mental space.

And what the future holds is not entirely in your hands yet, so cross that bridge when you come to it. Any negative thoughts that you may be harboring need to go as well for these will always hold you back.

Build a Positive Skillset

You need to do more than just exist; you need to live. Most people think that existing is enough simply because they have too much going on with not enough time to get it done in. It keeps them so busy that they can't really bother with things like simplification.

The problem with this scenario is that they miss out on the essence of life. To simplify means to indulge in a little bit of management. Manage your time and your life wisely so you develop a skillset of lifelong habits, organization, and punctuality.

As you simplify things when starting or stopping a habit, it can make execution a lot easier. For example, if you want to join a gym, choose one that is close to home. This will make it more convenient for you to go there every day easily. If you choose one that's far away, not only will you spend a lot of time getting there, you may stop sooner than planned because of the distance.

Likewise, keeping things simple can also teach you to become more organized. When you practice simplification, you learn how to manage things more efficiently.

This reduces the element of wastage and you not only learn how to save on costs but also how to improve your overall living standards.

And finally, when you complicate things, you also waste a lot of time. You overthink things that don't require attention and complicate them further.

Simplifying such matters teaches you punctuality and the importance of time. By keeping things simple you learn how to get them done well and on time.

CHAPTER 5

BE MINDFUL OF THE PRESENT

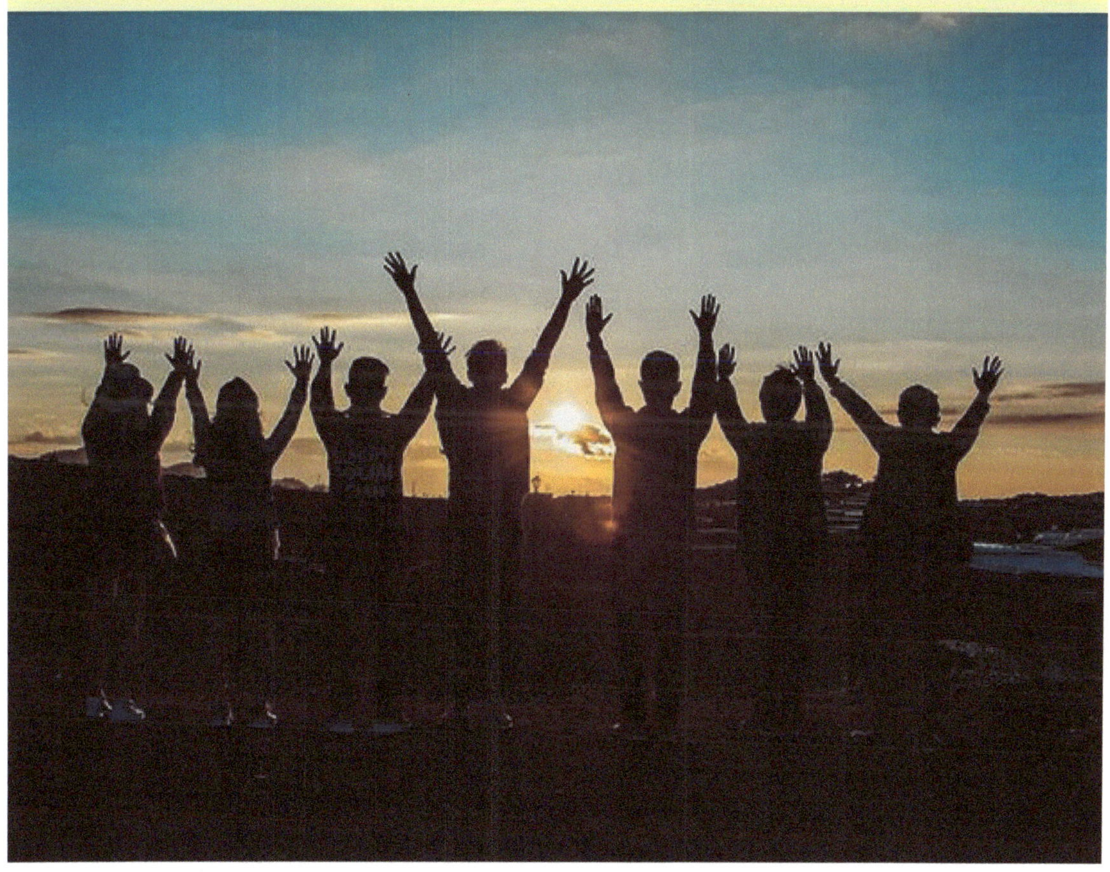

Chapter 5 - Be Mindful of the Present

Mindfulness is an ability that helps you recognize the happiness already present in your life. You don't have to wait years to find happiness. It is already there; you just have to see it.

Being mindful makes you realize that you are alive and breathing. It is when you are at peace with the present moment as it arrives. It may not be what you expected or wanted, but you are content with it.

This is perhaps one of the most important habits you'll need to infuse in your life if you want to make it more Zen-like. Because it lets you be content with who you are and what you have, it can easily be the happiest, most confident and safest place to be.

Plus, being mindful provides you hope that you can do so much more with life. By far it is the one solution that'll allow you to enjoy life to the fullest. The simple trick lies in not forgetting why something is important and doing it consciously.

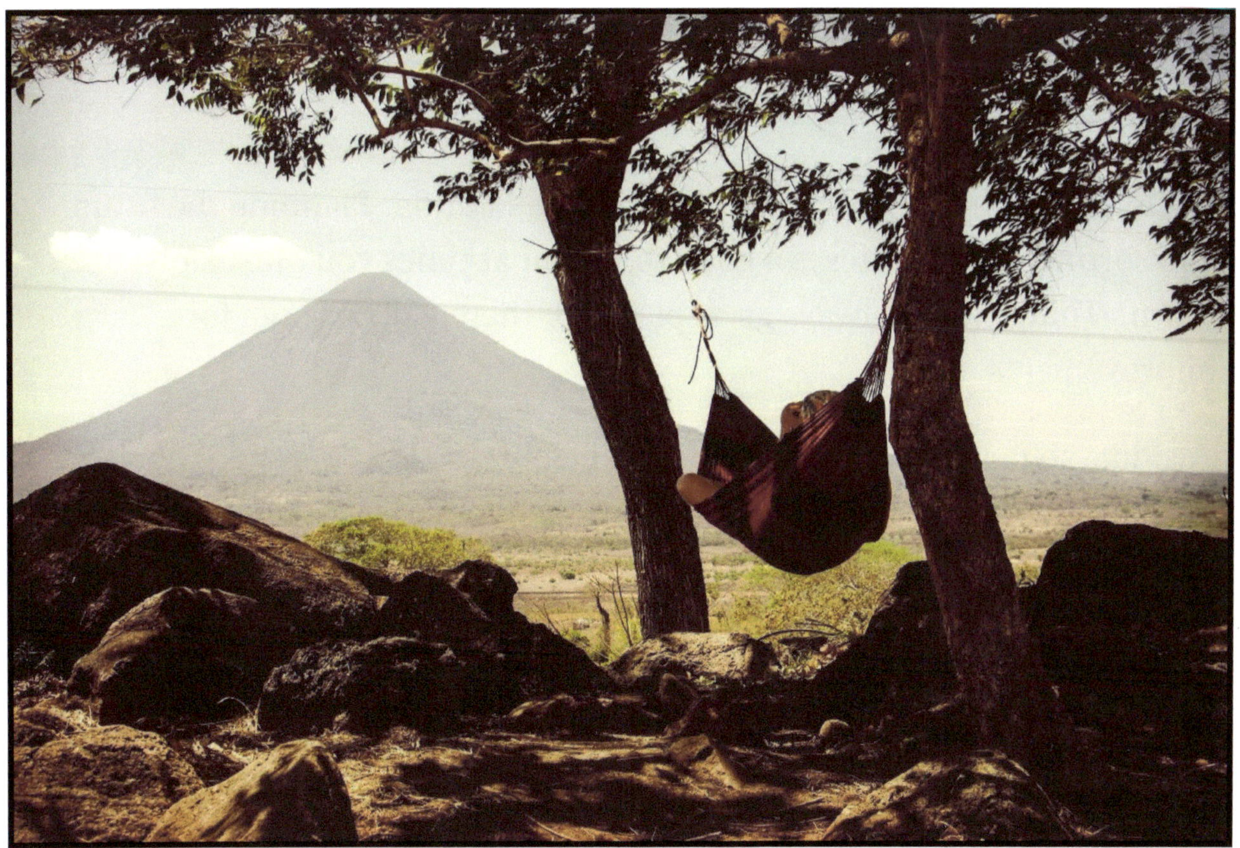

Most people have their minds stuck elsewhere. They simply move through the day without actually living it. This state is called forgetfulness. People stuck in this state can't develop focus or stay in the present. They are either busy thinking about the past or stuck in the future.

Mindfulness is the exact opposite of forgetfulness. Mindfulness means being there and living in the moment. A mindful state is one where you are mentally active. Your mind and the body are both in one place and this allows you to recognize happiness around you and feel it.

Being mindful doesn't require you to have special powers to stay awake. All that you must do is find joy in the little things.

Here's how you can learn to be a bit more mindful:

Slow Down

Rushing into things isn't always the perfect solution. Planning the future and sorting out activities is a good thing but at times you must slow down. Things won't always go as planned; there will be room for improvements.

Just like so many others, you may also be obsessed with speed. You want to be quicker, more efficient and more productive. To sum up, you just want to be faster.

Getting out of the habit of rushing and cramming things together can be particularly difficult if you want to step in the Zen zone.

This is because society rewards speed by career promotions, praise from peers and your belief that you're doing really well. Yet, despite all the rushing around, you don't really seem to be accomplishing anything extra. If anything, you get yourself more entangled into additional tasks, paying less and less attention to each.

And to top it all, rushing around doesn't help you perform any better. Instead, it will increase your stress levels and make you more disagreeable.

So take a moment and slow down. You'll notice that you enjoy life more. Things will seem more interesting and you'll have less to worry about.

Enjoy the Moment

Not everyone has the ability to enjoy moments especially when you don't get what you expect.

Say, you get stuck in a traffic jam, the price of gas skyrockets or you get an angry look from someone. All these experiences are disconcerting and some unnerving at best. So what do you do?

Most likely you compare the present moment with what you expect to happen. A traffic jam will get you late to work. The price of gas will upset your budget and you could spend the rest of your day wondering what you did wrong to deserve that angry look.

Sometimes you must give yourself room to breathe. Why complicate your life by focusing on things that don't really matter or are beyond your control? As my dad always said "Worry about the things you can control and not about the things you can't."

Instead, you can ease your life by enjoying what goes well. There are so many things in life that can provide happiness. All that is required on your behalf is the effort.

Many of us also miss out on life's precious moments simply because of stress. Life is unpredictable which is why it is important to live while you can.

For instance, you can find joy in the little things by learning to go with the flow. At times life exposes you to surprises that can be good or bad. To deal with these surprises you must go with the flow.

Going with the flow will let you engage in the reality of life. It's a Zen approach that lets you face what comes your way and you make a choice based on that. At the same time, it also means realizing that good and bad things happen in life and when they're beyond your control, you accept them as they come.

This way, you enable yourself to make the most of the moment despite any setbacks.

Another way of looking at this is that it lets you get past your failures. Accepting that you had a failure means that you face the reality of the situation. And based on that reality, you make choices to move forward.

If you never accept that reality, you'll get stuck at that point in time. You'll likely move forward without changing course and then the past will catch up with you once again. You'll get caught up in the spiral of past regrets and be in no position to enjoy the present.

Have Fewer Expectations

Expectations can lead to disappointment if things don't go the way you want them to. In this way, expectations can be extremely damaging to your happiness and put your happiness on hold.

Not to say that you shouldn't have expectations. It's just that you should have fewer expectations if you want to be happy.

That said, having realistic expectations lets you accept the flaws in people. But having unrealistic expectations will most often lead to disappointment.

You may have expectations from others as well as yourself. For instance, you may expect that when you work out and eat right, you'll get that perfect body. Or when you put in the extra hours, you'll get that promotion.

But when things don't pan out as you expected, you become frustrated, disappointed and angry with yourself and others.

Having fewer expectations lets you accept reality as it is. It also teaches you that your life can still be good without so many expectations. It is a humbling lesson that your life can be perfect as is without expecting it to be better.

Having fewer expectations will stop you from swaying up and down mentally based on whether good or bad things happen to you. Instead, you will no longer expect good or bad things to happen but just take them as they come. This means more contention for you and less disappointment.

When you stop judging things as good or bad, you'll feel lighter and have more freedom.

CHAPTER 6

MEDITATE A LITTLE EVERYDAY

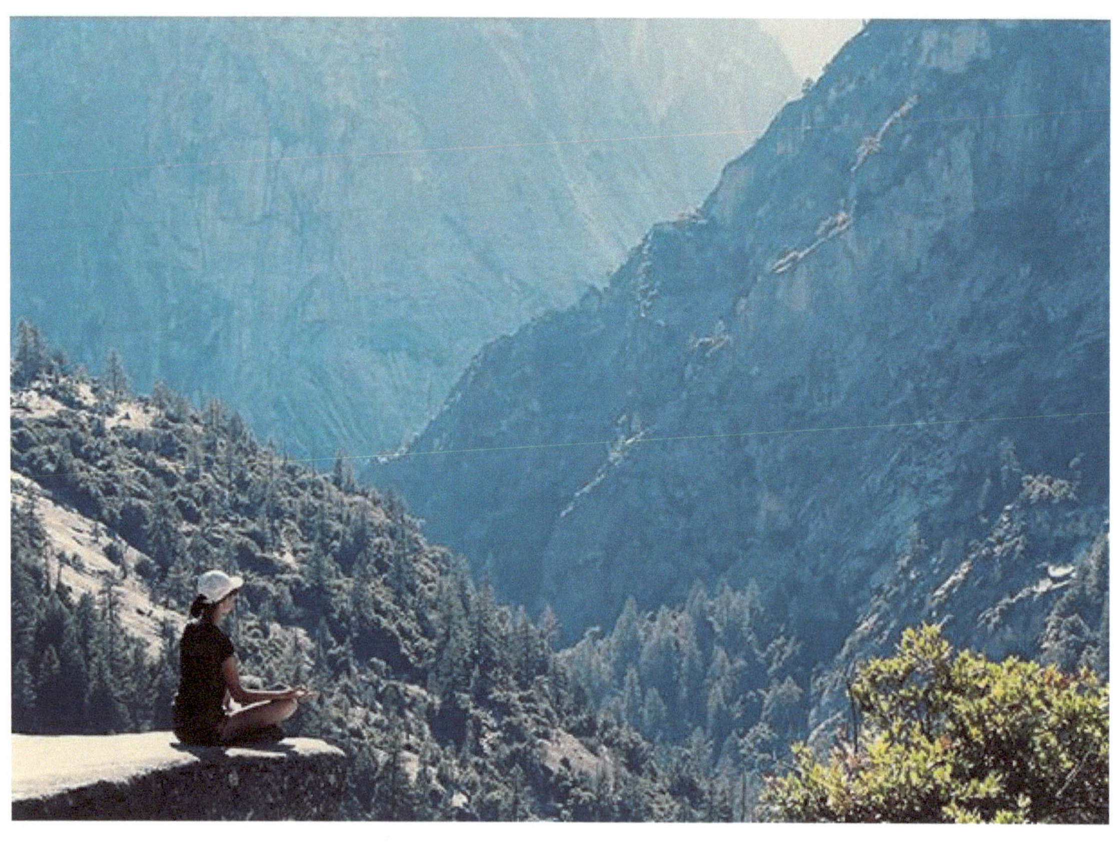

Chapter 6 - Meditate A Little Every Day

Meditation is an integral component of Zen habits. It is a long-established practice that helps you calm your mind, relax your body and focus on relaxation and stress relief. At its deepest level, meditation serves a spiritual purpose.

Zen meditation centers around a type of sitting meditation called zazen. The practice is all about sitting upright and following breathing.

Other types of meditation work around ideas of mental concentration on something – like a candle flame. Still others consider that meditation involves imagining a thing that gives you peace or satisfaction. In either scenario, the goal is to slow things down, especially the mind and stop its incessant activity.

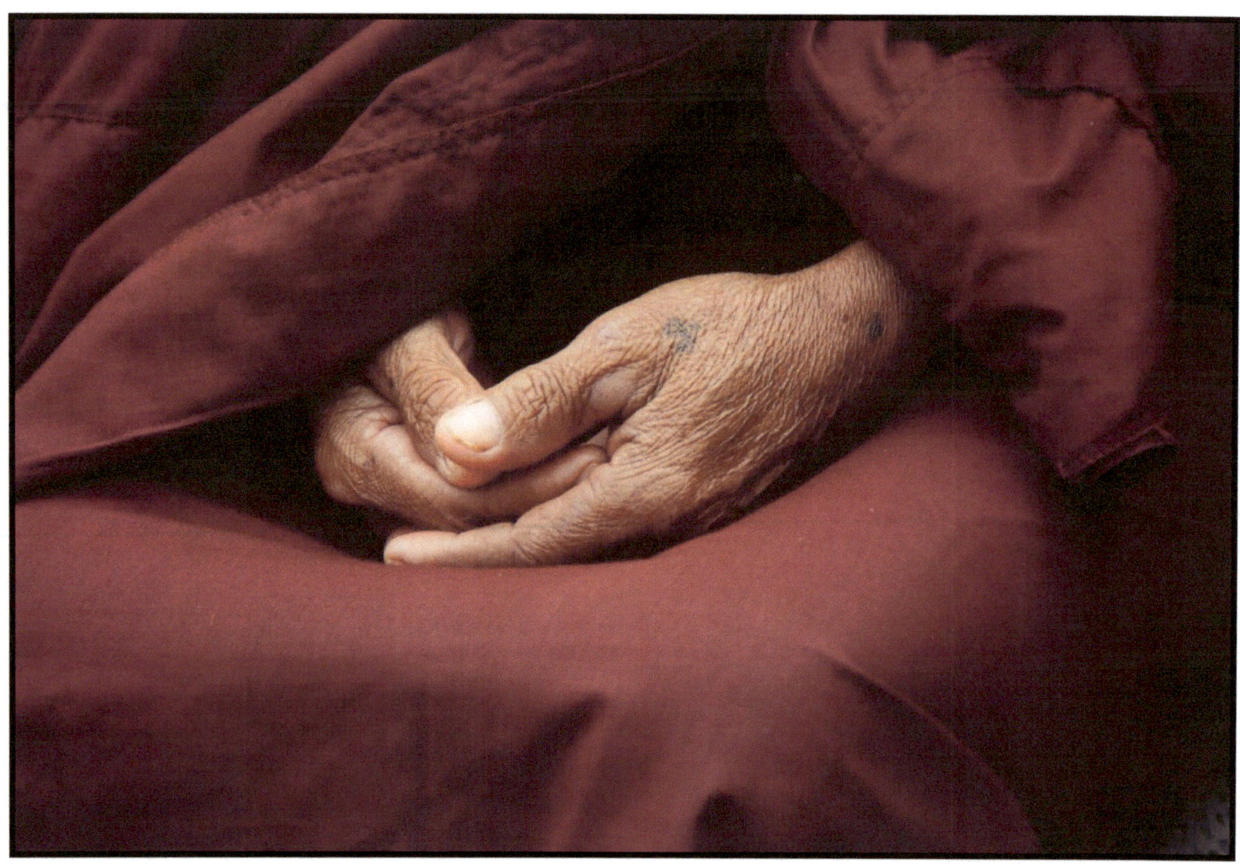

While Zen monks have known it for years, now science also backs up meditation as one of the most effective ways of dealing with stress. Although there are other stress reduction techniques present, this one by far is the most useful.

You can meditate for a number of different reasons. You can do so to develop concentration, clarity, or even emotional positivity. Depending on the type of meditation practice you follow, you can even learn the habits and patterns of your mind.

Most meditative states have a few basic commons. For instance, to enter a state of meditation, you will need to get into a relaxing position.

Choose a position that makes you feel comfortable but not too comfortable for you need to practice your focus. You can meditate sitting, standing, kneeling or even lying down. Certain forms of meditation will also let you sit in a chair and meditate.

Choose a posture that comes naturally to you. The key is to keep your back straight.

Entering a meditative state takes a few minutes. As you do this, keep your eyes closed and monitor your breathing. Breathing in and out cuts out distractions and lowers the heart rate.

Although there are many types of meditation, the focus here is on the main 3 types which are Yoga, Qigong, and Guided Visualization.

Let's have a look at each of these in detail:

Yoga

Yoga is a popular meditation technique that is practiced widely and is also considered a popular form of gentle exercises. Besides helping gain flexibility, strength, balance and even losing weight, yoga provides peace to the mind.

Most yoga poses require intent concentration which itself has a calming effect on the mind. This focus also helps reduce stress as your mind concentrates on your pose and not anything else.

As you maintain your pose, you also learn to control your breath which has a calming effect on the mind and body.

Although yoga isn't the complete cure for every ailment, it can benefit the human body in many ways. Yoga is the more cost-effective therapy for a better and happier life.

Some of the physical benefits of Yoga include:

- Improved stamina
- Improved flexibility
- Improved balance
- Increased strength

The mental benefits that yoga provides includes:

- Improved sleep
- Reduced stress
- Body awareness
- Improved state of mind

On a spiritual level, yoga aims to help you achieve a complete state of being. Advanced yogis can develop inner strength that gives them complete control over their emotions and desires. On the inside, it enables them to resist temptations and worldly pleasures.

If you reach an advanced level, you may also be able to learn to increase your self-esteem by practicing yoga. Removed from the worries of the world, yogis can experience the truth better and start to value themselves more.

Qigong

The second type of meditation technique is Qigong (pronounced chee-**gong**). This method helps improve posture and allows you to relax with ease. It is one of the oldest forms of meditation practiced by the Chinese.

Qigong consists of internal and external movements. This technique primarily involves the use of breath to circulate energy around the body.

There are a few different types categorized as moving, still and sitting meditation.

Moving meditation with Qigong involves the fluctuation of energy through postures, movements, breathing patterns and transitions. Postures that are held for long periods of time fall under still meditation while sitting meditation focuses more on the breath, body and mind.

The movement that is done in qigong promotes natural energy.

One branch of qigong known as medical qigong is part of Traditional Chinese Medicine. It's used to promote self-healing, disease prevention and addresses illnesses. The second known as martial qigong emphasises physical skill. This type lets practitioners demonstrate physical feats like breaking bricks and bending steel wires.

The third type known as spiritual qigong uses meditation practices and prayers to pursue enlightenmcnt.

When you use it for meditative purposes, qigong can help your body establish a relationship with the soul and mind. The method allows you to develop deeper spiritual development, body confidence and attention span.

Yoga and qigong are similar in quite a few ways as both contribute towards improved mental health.

Guided Visualization

Guided visualization is a type of relaxation technique that involves creating an image of a peaceful setting in the mind. This method is usually practiced in isolation as it requires a fair bit of focus and concentration.

You are encouraged to create a detailed mental image of a serene and attractive setting. The peaceful visual image is used to associate with the sensation of relaxation to calm the mind and body.

Guided visualization is also practiced with physical techniques such as a massage or progressive muscle relaxation. The aim is to make sure that the mind enters a state of peace.

The imagery used is used as a distraction tool to ward the mind away from things that may be stressing you. You may receive verbal or non-verbal instructions to let your mind relax.

Practicing this method requires both concentration and imagination. It cannot be practiced in noisy environments as interruptions easily put you off track and getting back into your tranquil state will be a lot more difficult.

This method plays a huge role in improving concentration abilities as focus is what is required. It also impacts cognitive abilities and improves memory power.

Guided visualization will require you to think better without a clogged mind. The technique will improve your creativity and promote peaceful thinking. When unwanted thoughts disturb your thinking process, guided visualization can help you get rid of them.

People seek this method because it allows them to relax. Finding peace can be a difficult thing but creating it on your own is easy. With guided visualization, you can promote inner peace by building a peaceful environment.

Meditation is the ultimate Zen habit to incorporate in your day. It might seem complicated but once practiced can turn your life around.

CHAPTER 7

ESTABLISH A DAILY ROUTINE

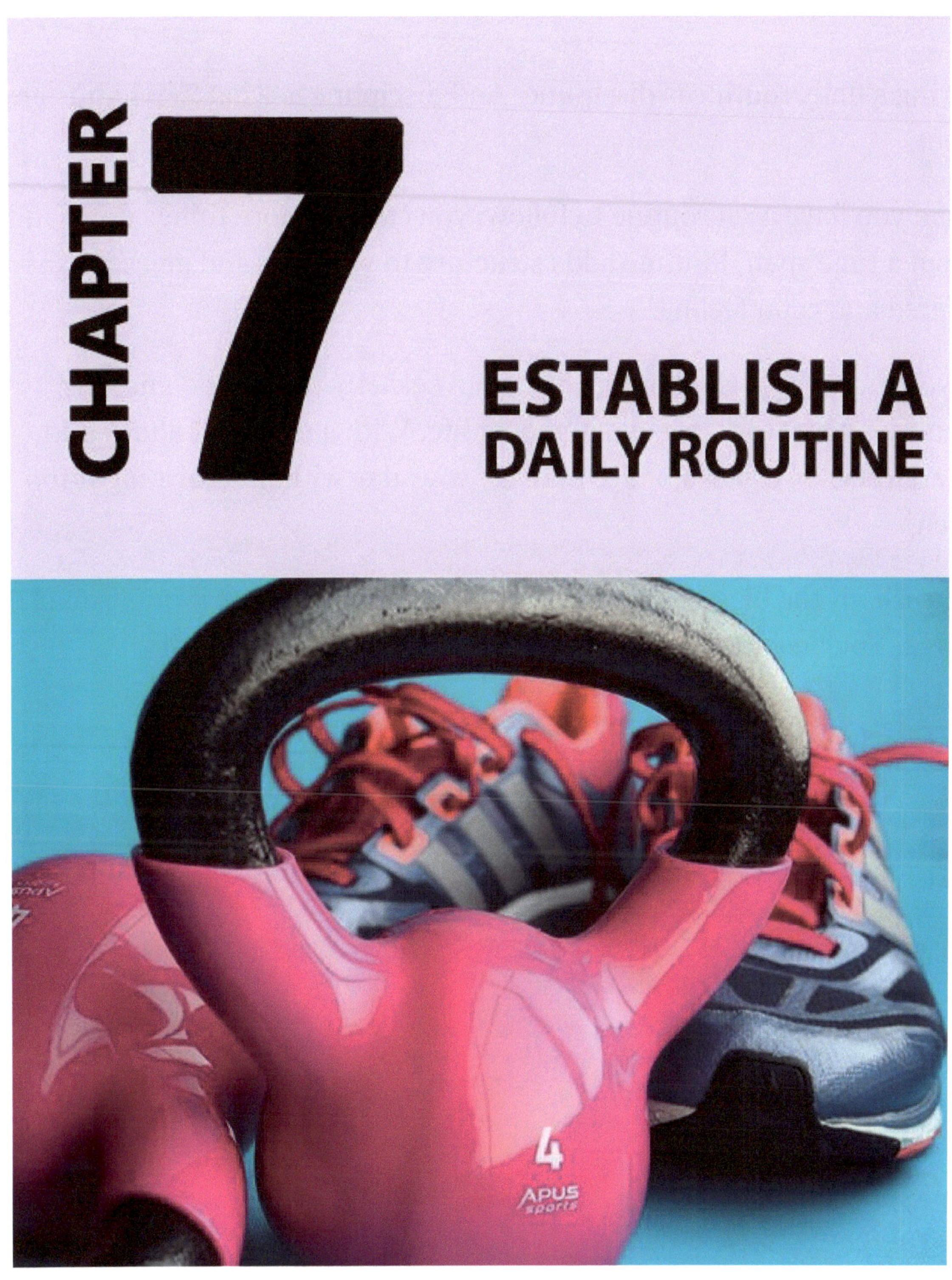

Chapter 7 - Establish a Daily Routine

Having a daily routine is discipline. And discipline is what Zen habits are all about.

When you have a set routine to follow, you can get more things done and in less of a time span. Routine adds structure to your day and gives it a more ordered and calm feeling.

As you move through your day, you know exactly what to do and this simplifies your work day and personal life. With a time-slot allotted to different tasks, you can better manage your day without crowding it too much.

But perhaps the biggest benefit of having structure is that it puts you in charge. You decide what's important and needs attention first.

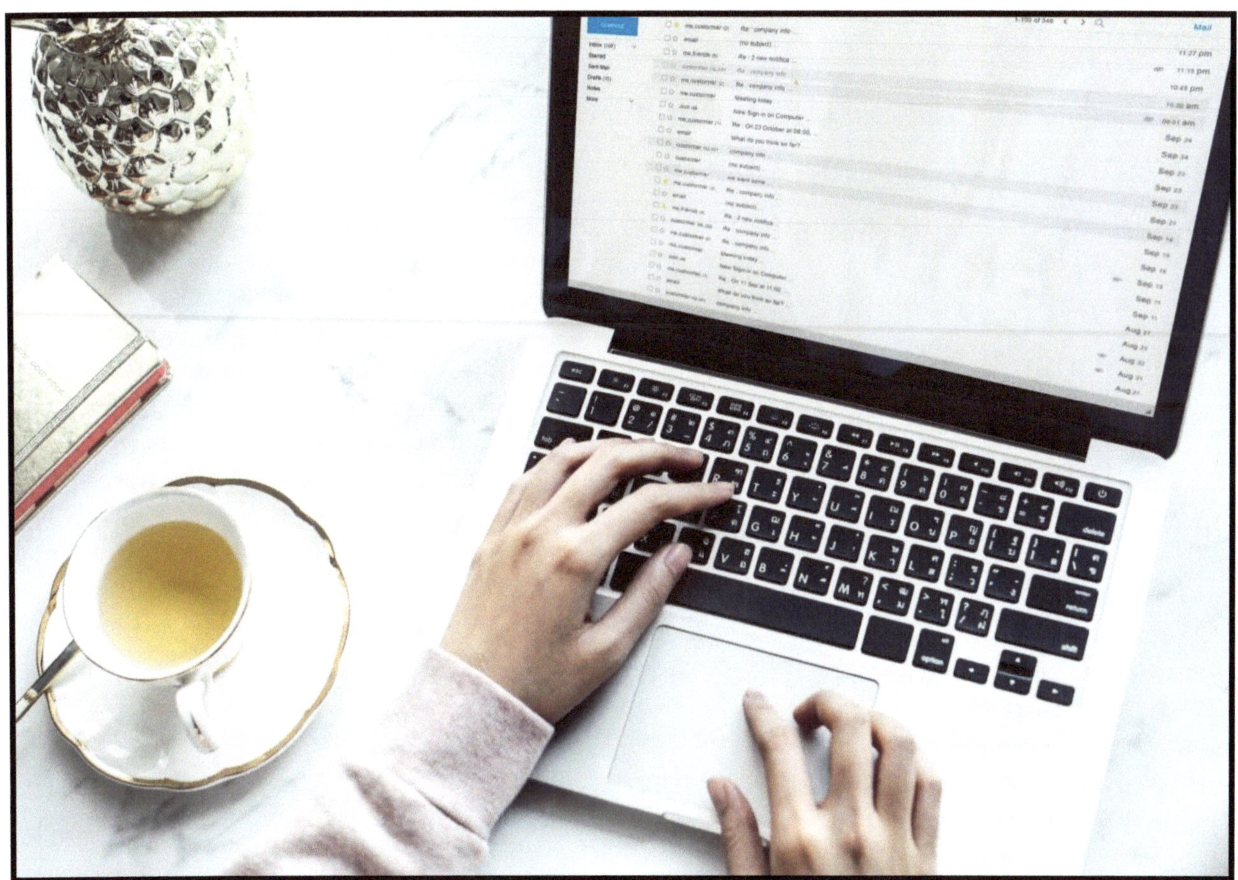

To make things easier you can divide up your routines into daily and weekly tasks. If you're able to stick with these for at least one month, they'll become lifelong habits.

It's not only planning your daily and weekly chores that need attention, but also how you take care of yourself during this time. You also need to establish healthy habits as part of your routine so you can take care of your body and mind in order to keep up with your planned schedules.

How do you do that? You pay attention to these aspects of your daily life.

Eating Well

You know that you have to eat healthy, but do you also know how to do it? This is the point where many people get lost as they're not sure how to implement this knowledge into action. But there is a simple way of doing this.

You may question what the connection between a set routine and eating is. Your eating habits define your lifestyle. If you eat clean and healthy you will have a better life and improved health. When you eat healthy you can function better and become more energetic.

Your starting point for eating well should be meal preparation. You can't go anywhere without this step. This will give you a fairly good idea of what you'll eat and what you'll have to stay away from. This step also involves shopping beforehand so that you have everything with you when you start cooking.

Moving on, you should build your meals around really healthy foods. Of course, you can have some wiggle room for slight indulgences, but the core of your eating plan should be based on super healthy stuff.

Make it a point to include foods that you really enjoy. This is very important if you want to eat well for the rest of your life.

The reason why so many diets fail is because they center on foods not everyone likes. If you can't/don't eat what you like, you won't stick with it for long. While anyone can follow a restrictive diet for a few weeks at most, if you start to feel deprivation and suffering, you'll give it up quickly.

So, the key to eating well all the time is to choose healthy and enjoyable foods. You can also add in variety and mix up the plan every now and then. But the key is to stay with foods you love.

Another aspect is food preparation. Keep your recipes simple for you don't want to be slaving over the stove endlessly. Choose meals that are quick to prepare and use fewer ingredients. This way you'll save up on time as well as money.

Mind your portion size as you eat. If you're eating healthy, nutritious foods, then you won't have to go in for seconds and thirds. What you eat in one serving should be enough to last you till your next meal.

Exercise

When establishing a daily routine, it is important that you make exercise a part of your routine. Exercise not only keeps you fit but also keeps you happy and has a mind-calming effect. It can even act as therapy for some.

In general, people who exercise tend to be more active and happier than those who don't. But it may not be the easiest habit to stick to.

Oftentimes, people start out exercising with a lot of energy and enthusiasm. They tell themselves, they'll run for 30 minutes every day or that they'll hit the gym daily. But the problem with this is that such a goal becomes too hard to sustain for long. You may be able to do it for a few days but then you burnout and the whole thing becomes a drag.

You may also tell yourself that you'll workout, eat healthy, quit desserts and go cold turkey on the soda all at the same time. This approach also creates problems because there are too many goals to deal with all at once.

Instead, what works in making exercise a regular part of your day is to start simple. Keep your exercise sessions short and simple in the beginning.

Decide on a time that'll work best for you. This way you're more likely to follow through and not put things off.

Start off with a 15-20 minute session and stick with it for at least two weeks. As your body gets used to exercising, you can then start prolonging your sessions and adding more intensity. But try not to up the duration and the intensity at the same time.

As you exercise, make sure that it's something you enjoy. As in the previous point, if you don't enjoy what you eat, you'll give up healthy eating altogether. The same goes for exercise. If you don't enjoy what you do, you'll stop doing it.

Remember that recovery is an important part of exercise. You may not need to have a rest day if you're only working out lightly for 20 minutes or so. But as you progress towards more advanced sessions, make sure to add in rest days to give your body a chance to recover … at least one day per week.

On your rest days, indulge in some very light exercise such as going out for a walk. The point is to never actually skip a day as this makes creating a habit more difficult. Do something that keeps you moving, even though very slightly. This will keep your habit formation going.

Lower Stress

While a stress-free life is really not possible, you can try and lower your stress levels considerably. It's possible because many of the things you stress about are unnecessary.

For most people stress stems from things like meeting deadlines, dealing with difficult people, job uncertainty, competition, conflicts, not enough time and an overall sense of being swamped by too much. When things get out of control you start to stress out.

If you want to lower stress levels from your life, then you need to have some sort of a method to do so. For instance, you need to recognize the signs of stress. When you feel the stress coming on, pause and take notice.

You may feel this as a physical sensation of rushing and crashing down. Or may recognize it as a headache coming on. Whatever the signs, you need to stop and slow down. If you feel that you're not in control any longer, just stop doing whatever is bringing on this feeling.

You need to recognize that you can't be in control all the time so don't let it get the better of you. Know that you can't do everything at once, so pick and choose your tasks wisely. Narrow your scope to bring things in perspective and renegotiate your commitments.

Choose only what is doable and focus on one thing at a time. As you fully give yourself to that one thing, feel the tension melt away and relax into the moment. Accepting what's going on will make you better at lowering stress than trying to fight it.

If people bring you stress, shy away from them and stay with others who make you feel good. If things get in the way, seclude yourself and meditate, stretch, massage or get some fresh air until you are ready to face the challenges again.

Schedule to take mini-breaks every day to destress on a continual basis. This is the only way to charge yourself again for the next onslaught of the daily grind.

CHAPTER 8

RESPECT AND APPRECIATE LIFE

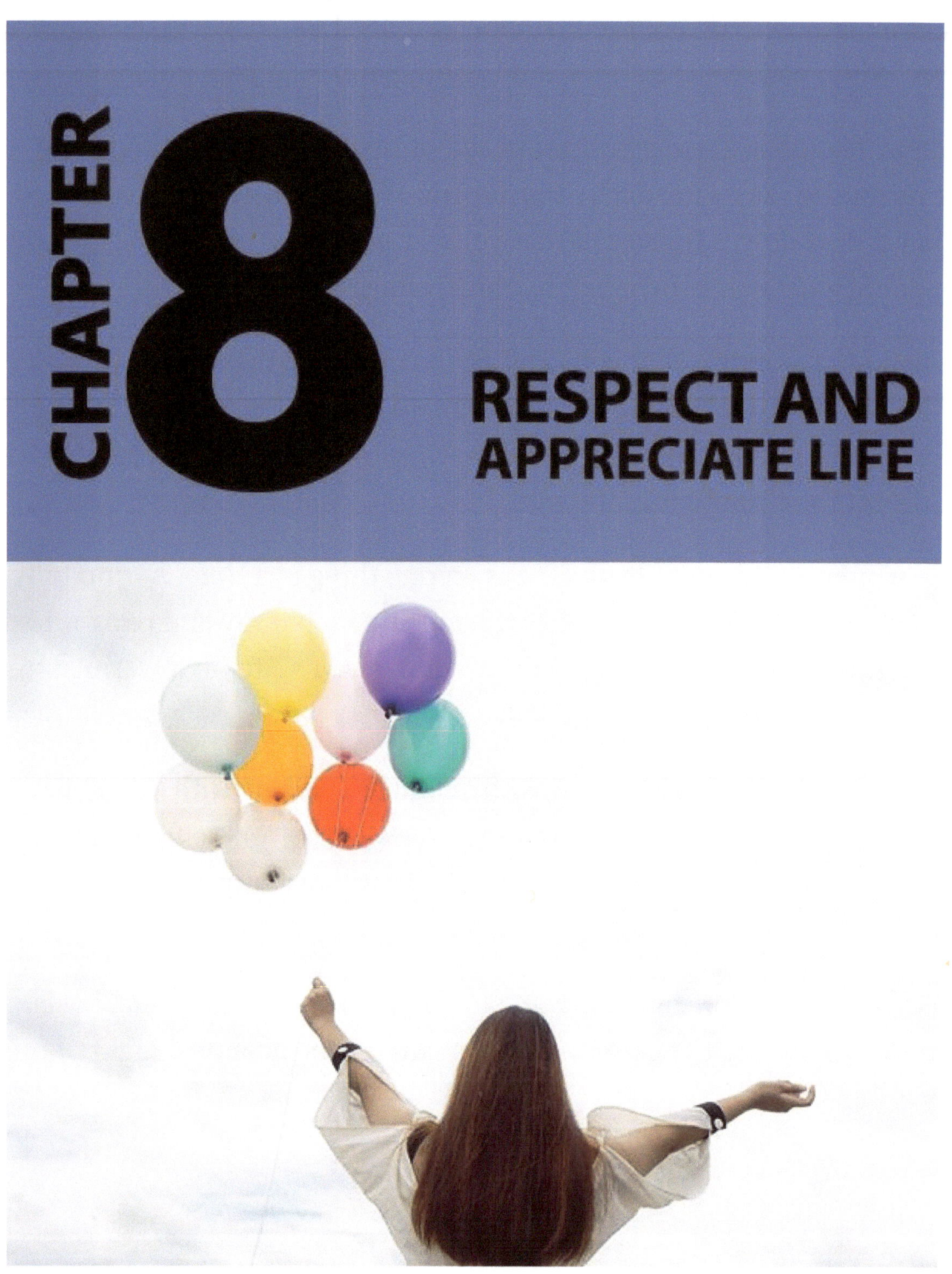

Chapter 8 - Respect and Appreciate Life

People who can find happiness in small things are those who live a happy life.

For others, it's easy to forget what they have since they're so busy looking for what they don't have. It's funny how the mind works- thinking that what you could have will be more valuable than what you do have. But just how do you measure this happiness?

There are people who have a lot of money but aren't happy and then there those who have no money but are happy. This difference exists because of their state of mind. Those who appreciate life find happiness no matter what.

While happiness itself can mean a lot of different things for different people, those who are the happiest may not necessarily *have* the best of everything. But they do *make* the best of everything.

If your happiness is associated only with achieving certain goals such as a nice car or a good job, then rest assured that the search for happiness will be a lifelong pursuit. This is because once you get these goals, you look forward to meeting more goals which will make you happier and so on. In other words, your happiness is always placed somewhere in the future, but never in the present.

On the contrary, happy people are always happy in the present. Their happiness is right here and now with who they are and what they're doing. They learn to appreciate life as it and don't give a thought to how great things will be in the future.

If you want to lead a happier life, try including these Zen habits to appreciate life better.

Learn To Let Go

This may sound difficult to do but learning to let go can release you from a lot of worries. At times you stick on to things that don't matter. You feel that if you let go you won't be able to survive.

In essence, it's an attempt to hold on to meaningless issues for more meaningful ones. When letting go you need to realize that walking away from certain situations is a step forward. In fact, there are times when certain things in your life aren't meant to stay.

Perhaps the most difficult part about letting go is moving out of your comfort zone and into new territory. But remember that change happens for a reason and you should be ready to embrace it.

Consider the example of a couple who splits. Either way, both parties involved will be impacted but until and unless they let go, can't they reduce the impact.

Holding onto pain or unpleasant memories doesn't fix anything. If anything, it holds you back. It could be a tragedy, or an untimely death leaving you pining for what could've been. You yearn for what should've been or what you feel you were entitled to.

It could also be a dream, a desire, a hope or a wish. Something that you may have wanted for years but never actualized.

It becomes very important to let go because all this is dead weight. And the longer you hold onto it, the longer it takes for you to move forward.

The same also stops you from investing in your present and being happy at the moment.

Even when you look at all the stuff you possess ask yourself- do you really need to have so many things?

That shirt you stopped wearing ages ago still hangs in your closet. Those shoes that were your best friend in your college days still have a spot on the shoe rack. And all those books which you'll never open again are taking up half the bookshelf. You talk about letting go but keep holding onto excess baggage.

Learn to let go of things and let more life in.

Turn More to Nature

There is no denying the fact that everyone feels happier when they are in nature.

Mother Nature never disappoints and always provides inner peace. Being in nature helps reduce stress levels and if you notice, time also slows down when you're in nature.

The sense of urgency and rush that you experience in your daily life seems to come to a standstill when you turn to nature. Instead it's replaced by a healthier pace of life. Things in nature happen according to their natural rhythm instead of being dictated by clock time.

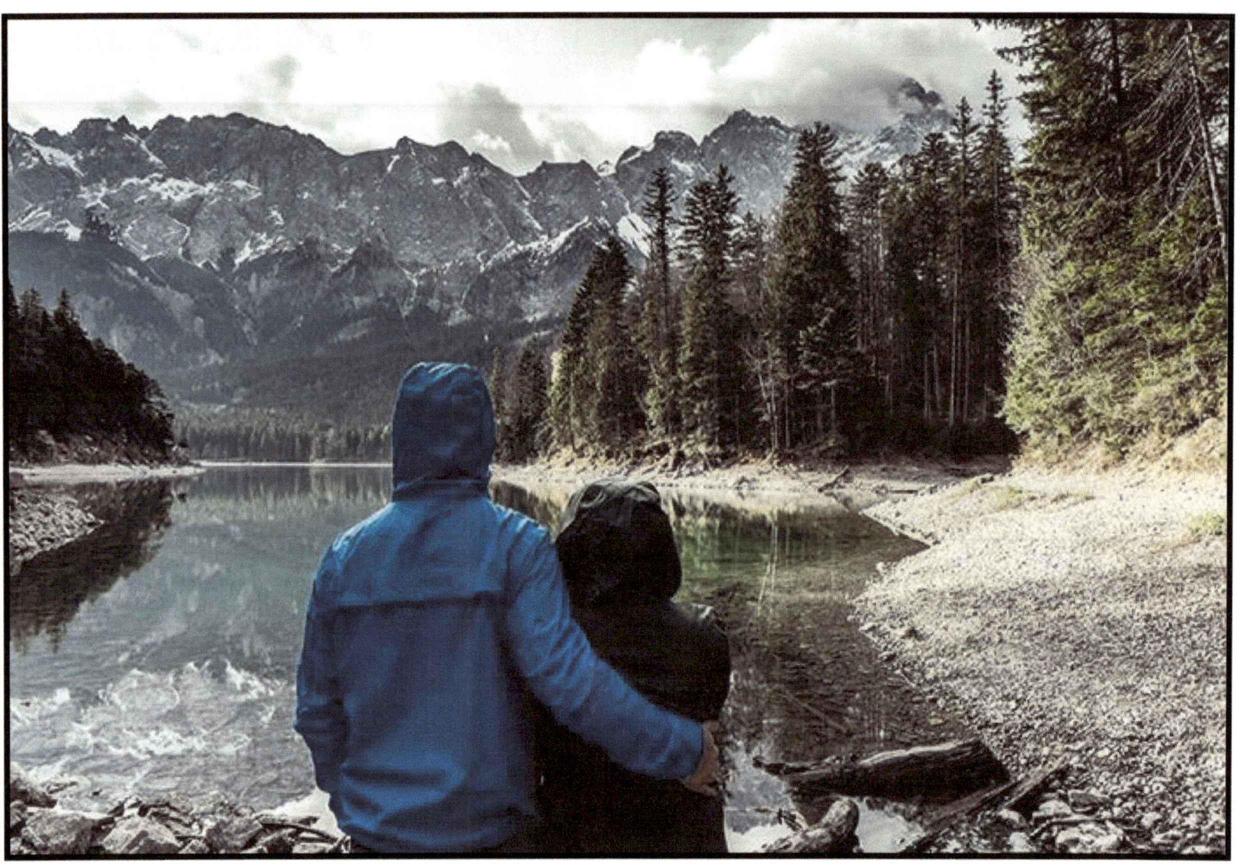

When you spend more time in nature, you stop to enjoy the scenery and learn to appreciate more. You learn to breathe slowly and relax and get relief from the daily grind. It is possibly one of the best ways to add more Zen into your life.

When you cut yourself off from nature, you get assimilated by the drive to be as comfortable as possible, to make your life as pleasurable as possible and to resist as much hardship as you can. But the truth is that you can never be pleased or comfortable all the time. And you certainly can't always be in control.

Staying in touch with nature brings you back to reality. So many things in nature are beyond your control such as the rising and setting sun. You can't control when it rains or when the temperature gets too high. You learn to accept these elements as they are which is a lesson in humility.

It makes you realize how little control you really have. You accept this reality and learn to be happy in your given situation.

Happiness Is Closer Than You Think

To conclude, the quest for happiness doesn't have to be an impossible task. It's right there for you to behold, if you choose to do so.

Contrary to popular opinion which looks for happiness in nicer things, you can find happiness in the simplest of things. Have a productive day, go out for a walk in nature, or listen to a beautiful song. Notice how all these unspectacular things can make you happy. All you need to do is connect with happiness and it'll be right there for you.

Happiness isn't something that you can get from external things but comes from within you. It is also not something that happens to you but something that you make happen. And remember that you'll never find happiness if you keep looking in the wrong places.

To look for happiness outside yourself stops you from being yourself. So instead of searching for happiness, just be yourself and you'll find that happiness will come to you.

Some people experience a sense of happiness through giving. This is because giving connects you with others. So, if that's where you feel happy, then give away generously.

You may also have reminisced over the past thinking about those "happier days". But if you think hard enough and try to remember why were you happy at the time that you now consider to be a happier time? You'll probably realize that you never took note of your happiness as you experienced it. This is because in your mind happiness is something that lives in the memory rather than something you consciously experience.

To associate happiness with either the past or the future leaves no room for it in the present.

This is what you must change. Focus on gratitude and count your blessings so you can learn to be happy in the moment. Chances are you already have happiness in your midst but just don't realize it.

Conclusion

A Zen lifestyle means you must filter, weed, eliminate and edit a lot of habits, possessions, mindsets and perspectives from your life. All this is to simplify and minimize your life to make it a more purposeful existence.

It is a fight against speed and time, where you get yourself out from the constant swirl of unending worries and thoughts. You slow down the pace of your daily life, remove all that isn't necessary and enjoy life as it comes your way. Try these Zen habits and see how much better you'll feel and at peace with yourself.

As a thank-you for purchasing this book, be sure to get our report ***5 Zen Principles for a Better Life*** free. Download it at: https://forms.aweber.com/form/76/1111507776.htm.

About the Author

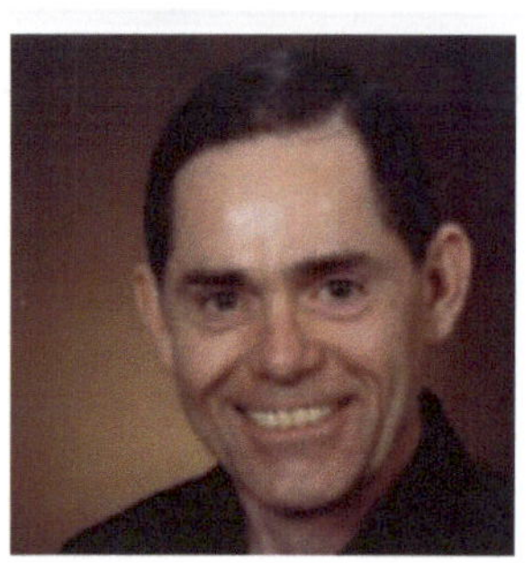

I grew up in Central Minnesota, where my parents owned and operated a fishing resort. Once out of high school I tried a couple of semesters of college, only to quit halfway through the Spring term; I decided at that time that college wasn't for me.

Then I decided to follow my father's previous occupation as an auto mechanic. I graduated from a two-year of vocational training course and worked as a mechanic for five years. While in vocational training, I decided to join the National Guard where I eventually ended up working full-time for 32 years.

So how does all of this relate to writing? In one of my leadership schools, the instructor, who was an English teacher at a juvenile detention center, presented writing to me in a whole new way - a way that started to develop my interest in working with words.

I eventually went back to college on the GI Bill while I was working and earned my Bachelor's degree in Business Administration. Taking a class or two per semester at night and on weekends took me seven years to complete my degree.

Fast forward about 40 years and I now have published over 100 books on Amazon for Kindle, CreateSpace and other publishing platforms.

Besides my own writing, I also ghostwrite ebooks, books, reports, articles, blogs and do Kindle conversions for clients on a variety of topics.

Today my wife and I are retired from our careers and live in Gold Canyon, AZ. I now write as a retirement business where you'll find me happily sitting in my office typing away on my laptop as I work on my next book or ghostwriting project . . . that is if we are not traveling on a cruise ship - our new-found mode of travel.

Thank-you for purchasing this book. If you are interested in purchasing and reading more of my published books, you can go to https://www.amazon.com/Ron-Kness/e/B0072M6PYO.

www.ingramcontent.com/pod-product-compliance
Lightning Source LLC
Chambersburg PA
CBHW040134240726
48664CB00002B/473